OBSTETRIC ANAL SPHINCTER INJURIES MADE SIMPLE

Birth related perineal trauma (BRPT) and obstetric anal sphincter injuries (OASIS)

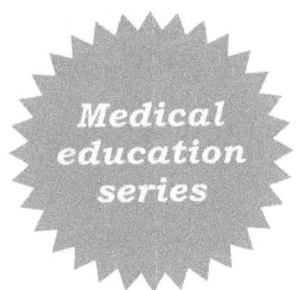

Medical education series

SSabri

Preface

The audience targeted include patients, this will also be useful for clinicians.

This will provide better understanding of anal sphincter complex, risk of injuries during normal and obstructed labor as well as collaboration and team working approach between uro-gynecologist, colorectal and midwife team.

Obstetric Anal Sphincter Injury (OASI) can have have long term implication leading to patients making the decision not to pregnant again or going forward for Cesarean section.

Anal incontinence and rarely rectovaginal fistula formation have an effect on quality of life (QOL)and relationship as well as feeling low in general. This will be an addition of existing literature to have a better understanding in simple language.

SSabri

Special Thanks

Muhammad Aamir
Areej and Areeb

Keywords for book

Anal Sphincter injury, anal incontinence, obstetrical complications, pregnancy, overlap repair of external sphincter injury, end to end repair of anal sphincter, laceration of perineum sphincteroplasty, pelvic floor conditions, obstructed labor, levator-Ani Avulsion, pelvic floor dysfunction.

Table of contents

Obstetric Anal Sphincter Injuries

Introduction

Approximately 1-3 % of women who deliver vaginally usually experience third and fourth degree vaginal tear

This involves the tissues of vagina, perineal area this area is around vagina and rectum, as well as structures around the anus

Obstetric anal sphincter injuries are most common of incontinence in child bearing age.

Many OASIS remain unrecognized and there is underreporting with incidence as low as 1-2 % of vaginal deliveries.

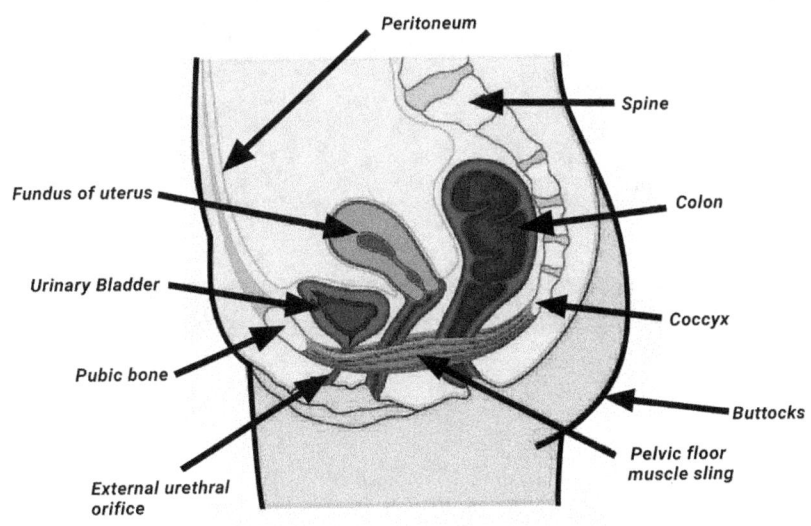

Sagittal View of pelvis Anatomy

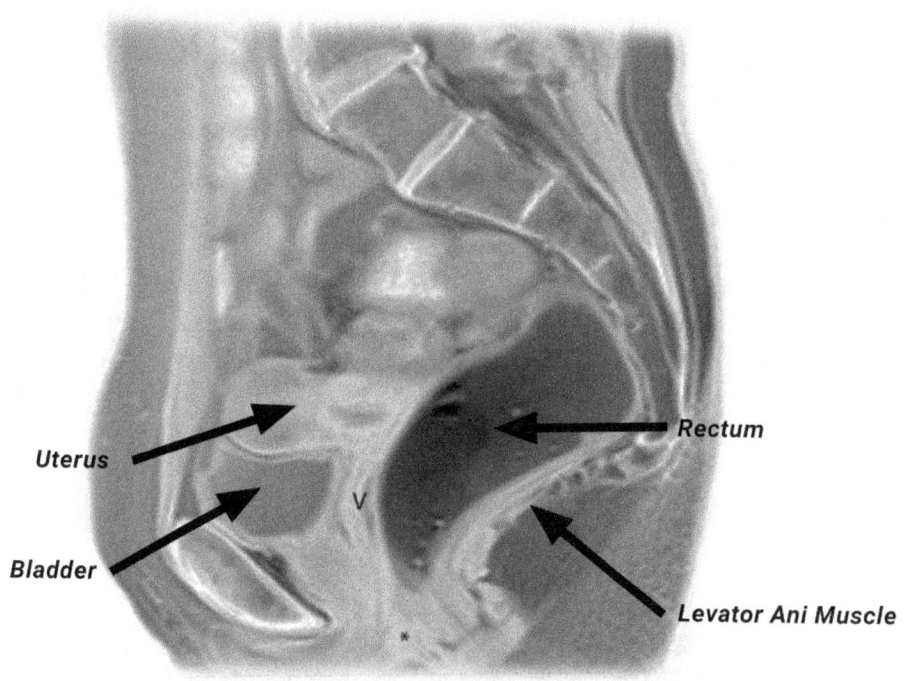

Uterus

Bladder

V

Rectum

Levator Ani Muscle

Sagittal View of pelvis Anatomy

When assessing for perineal trauma lithotomy or recumbent position is the preferred position.

Vaginal examination should be performed to assess for presence and extent of tear, the structures involved, apex of injury and assessment of bleeding.

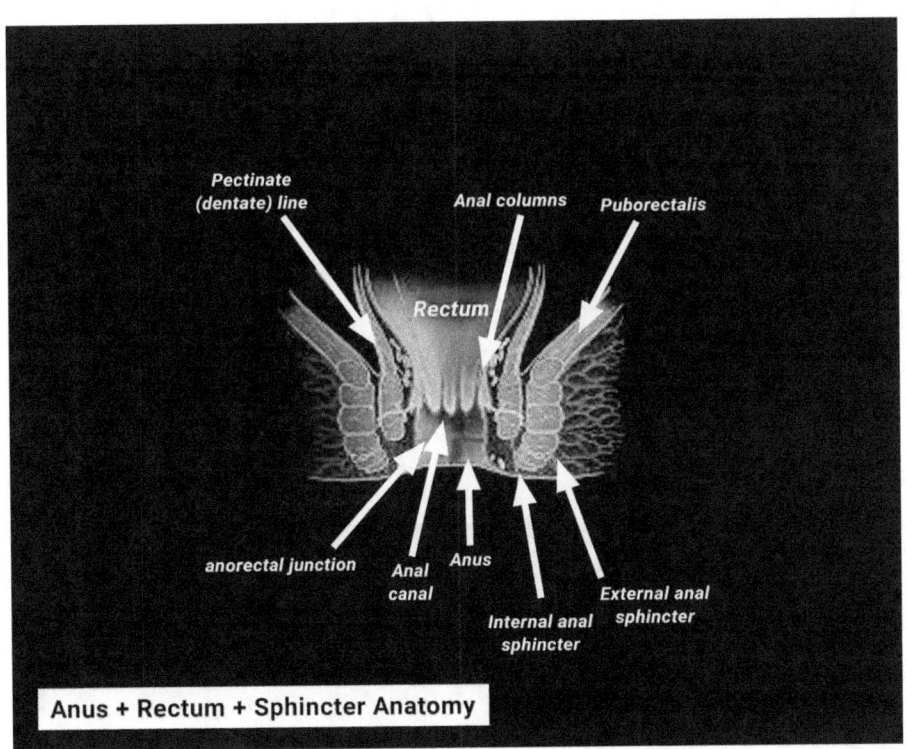

Anus + Rectum + Sphincter Anatomy

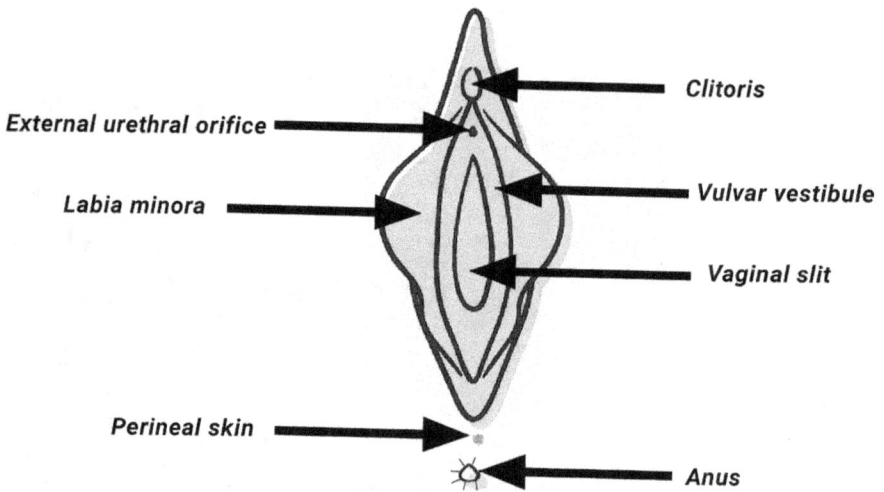

Clitoris

External urethral orifice

Labia minora

Vulvar vestibule

Vaginal slit

Perineal skin

Anus

Female Genital Anatomy

First degree	Injury to perineal skin only
Second degree	Injury to perineum involving perineal muscles but not involving the anal sphincter
Third degree	Injury to perineum involving the anal sphincter complex
3a	Less than 50% of EAS thickness torn
3b	More than 50% of EAS thickness torn
3c	Both EAS and IAS torn
Fourth degree	Injury to perineum involving the anal sphincter complex (EAS and IAS) and anal epithelium

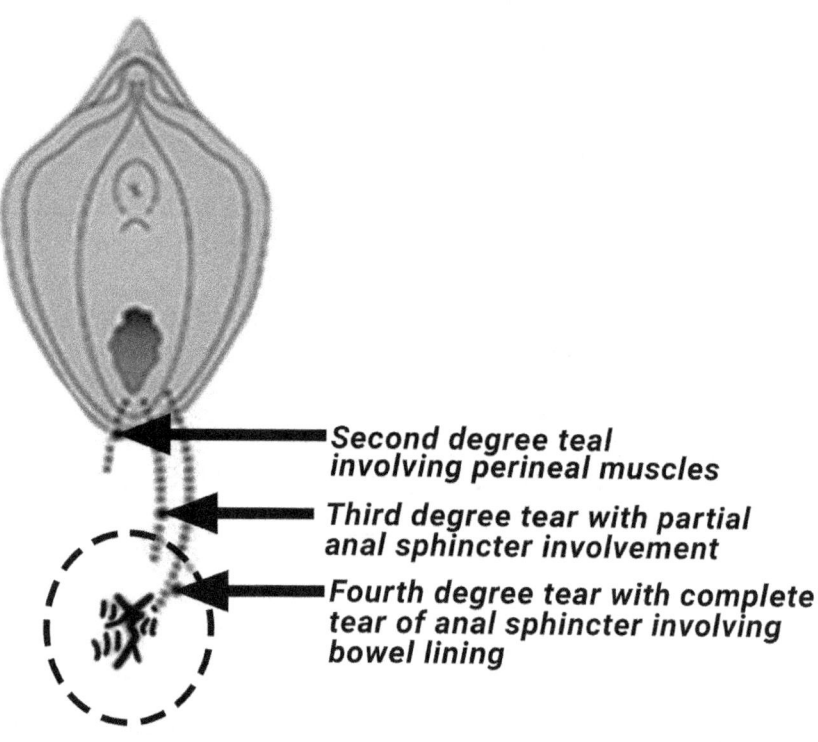

Second degree teal
involving perineal muscles

Third degree tear with partial
anal sphincter involvement

Fourth degree tear with complete
tear of anal sphincter involving
bowel lining

OASI diagrammatic presentation

First Degree

Injury to the perineal skin and vaginal mucosa.

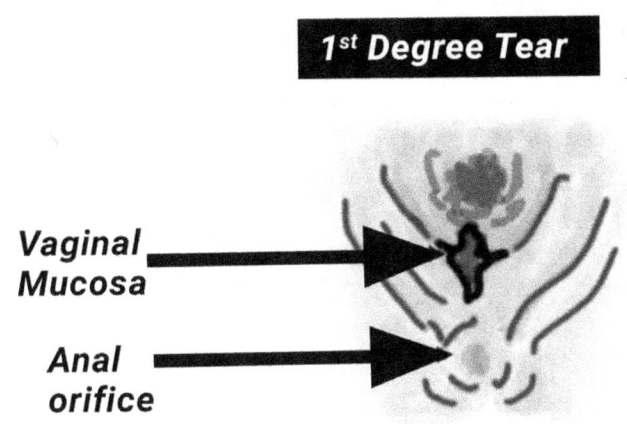

1st Degree Tear

Vaginal Mucosa

Anal orifice

Second Degree

Injury to the perineum involving the perineal muscles but not involving the anal sphincter

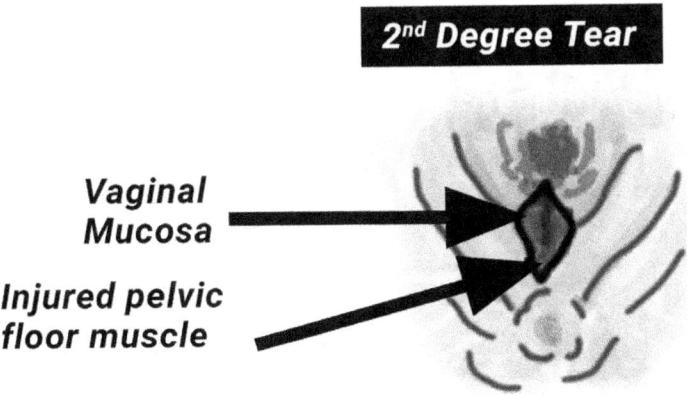

2nd Degree Tear

Vaginal Mucosa

Injured pelvic floor muscle

What is third degree perineal tear?

3rd degree tear involves partial sphincter fibres.

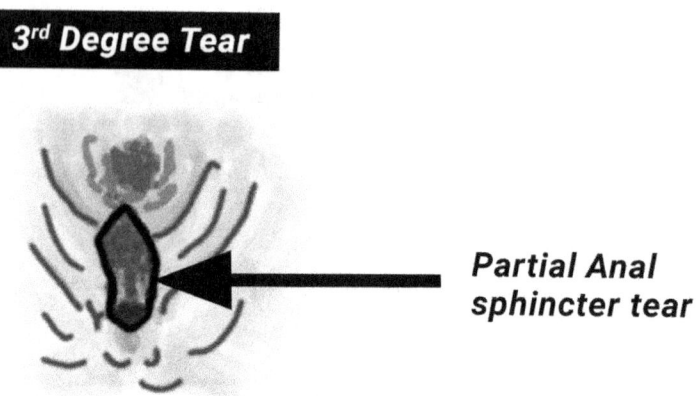

Partial Anal sphincter tear

What is fourth degree perineal tear?

4th degree tear involves complete tear of anal sphincter fibers.

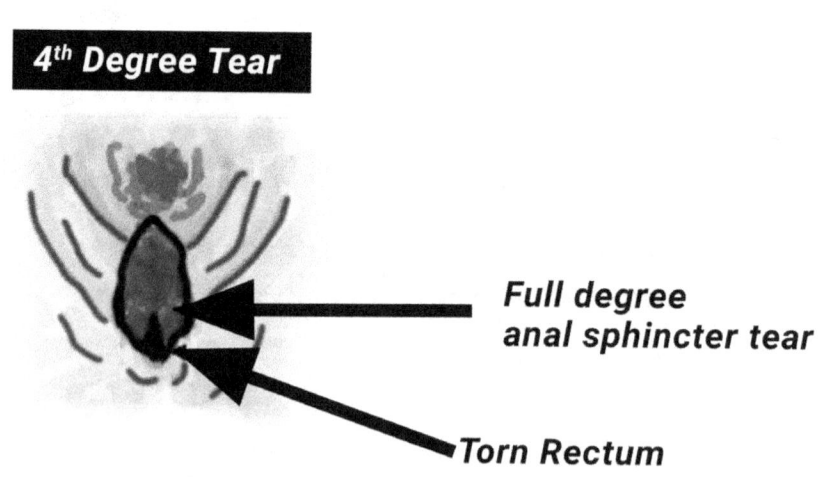

Full degree anal sphincter tear

Torn Rectum

Treatment of third and fourth degree tears?

These tears are repaired in the operating theater under local or general anesthesia. prophylactic antibiotics are given, the layer of tear will be stitched back together.

The stitches are dissolvable, and the urinary catheter is also placed until the effect of anesthesia is over.

Internal Anal Sphincter injury

Repair is performed end to end with interrupted 3-0 PDS sutures. The suture is monofilament and less likely to participate in infection. The internal anal sphincter IAS is responsible for maintaining continence at rest.

External Sphincter injury

1. Less than 50 % of injury (An end to end repair should always be performed with mattress suture to approximate the muscle ends).

2. When more than 50 % of EAS is torn (3 b) perform overlap repair. Overlap repair is not possible until the EAS is completely torn in length and thickness. Perineal suturing repair is audited against NICE standards and guidelines. Repair can be delayed for 8-12 hrs for experience. Repair of external anal sphincter should include the fascial sheath

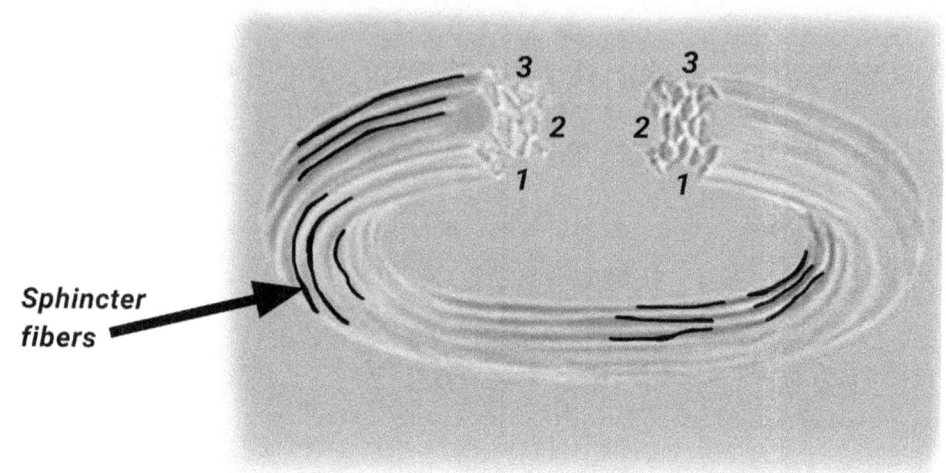

Mattress suture to approximate the muscle ends

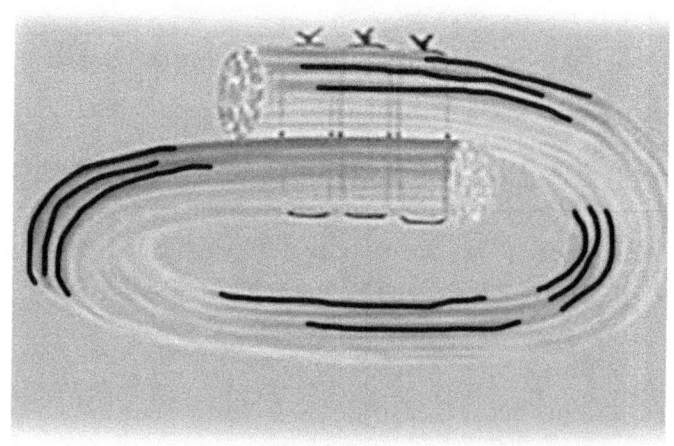

Overlap repair technique

PDS sutures are suitable to to be used to repair the sphincter fibers.

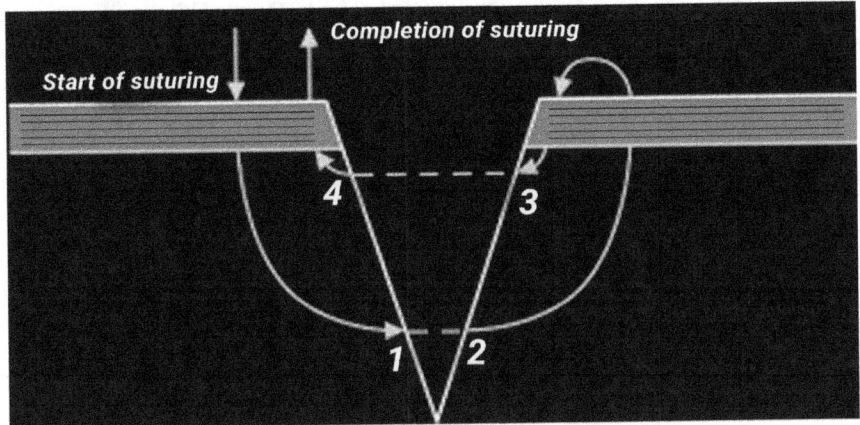

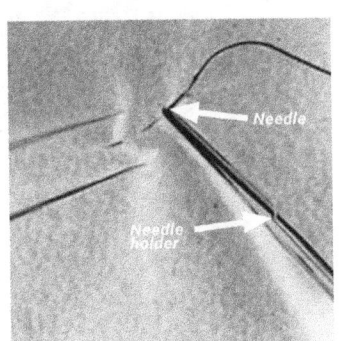

Head Control........
- Slowing down delivery of head and help of uterine expulsive movements decreases the incidence of oasis.

Perineal Support
- Application of warm compress the perineum as well as intrapartum perineal massage

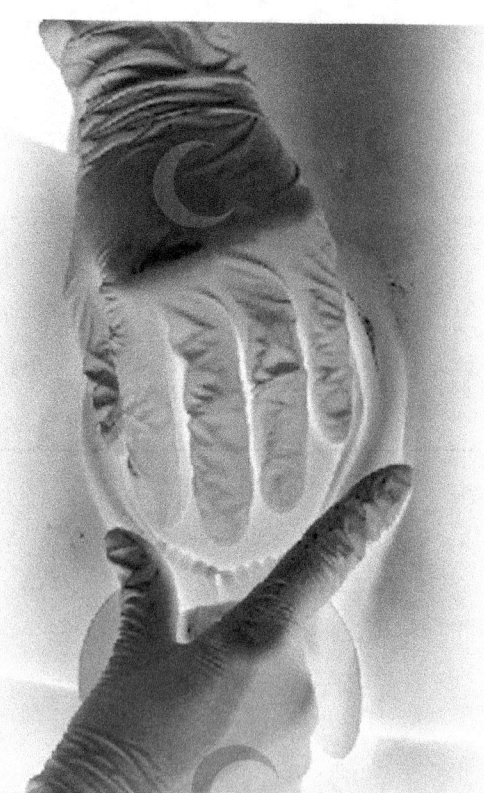

The perineal protection

Rectovaginal Fistula

- Rectovaginal fistula (RVF), defined as any abnormal connection between the rectum and the vagina, is a debilitating and complex condition

- RVF can occur for a variety of reasons, but frequently develops following obstetric injury.

- Patients with suspected RVF require thorough evaluation, including history and physical examination, imaging, and objective evaluation of the anal sphincter complex.

- Prior to attempting repair, sepsis must be controlled and the tract allowed to mature over a period of 3 to 6 months.

- Plugs are used for implantation to reinforce soft tissue for repair of recto-vaginal or anorectal fistulas.

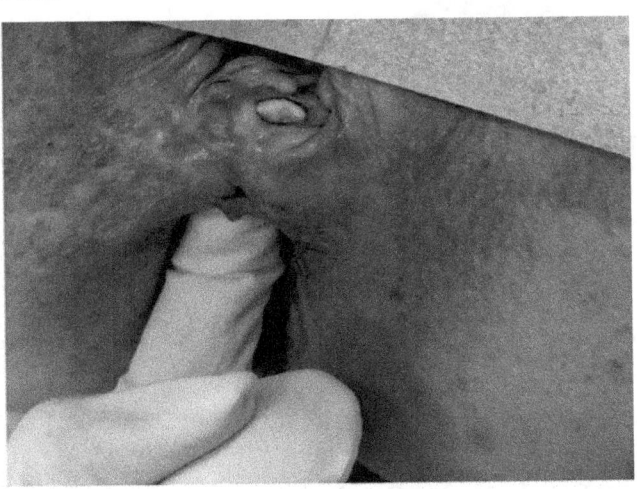

EUA (Examination under anaesthesia) digital examination to see the extent of recto-vaginal fistula , placing plastic cannula , blue dye , fistula probe all can be considered before considering the treatment options.

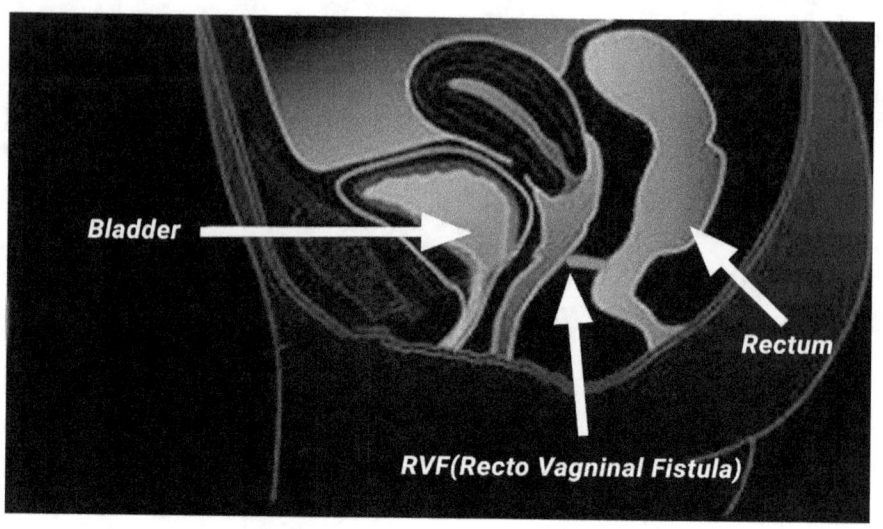

Bladder

Rectum

RVF(Recto Vagninal Fistula)

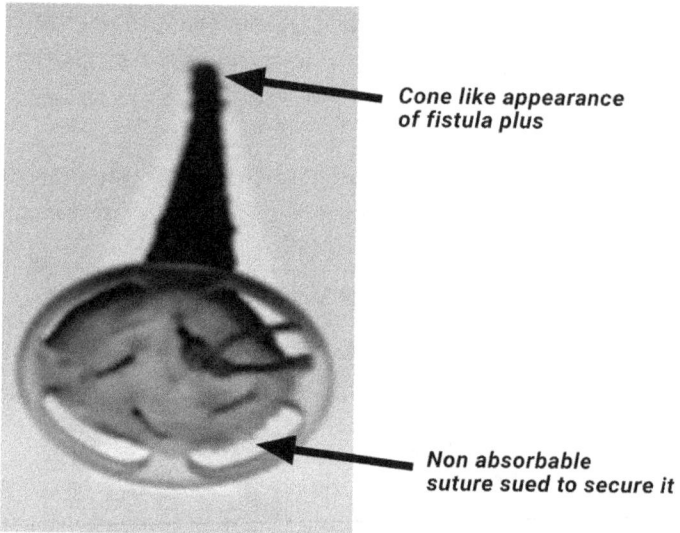

Cone like appearance
of fistula plus

Non absorbable
suture sued to secure it

Fistula plugs are cut , tailor made depending on the size of fistulous tract, for fistula in rectovaginalarea following the placement of probe is stitched on both sides with vicryl sutures. Patient are advised for not to have sex for short period of 6 to 8 weeks.

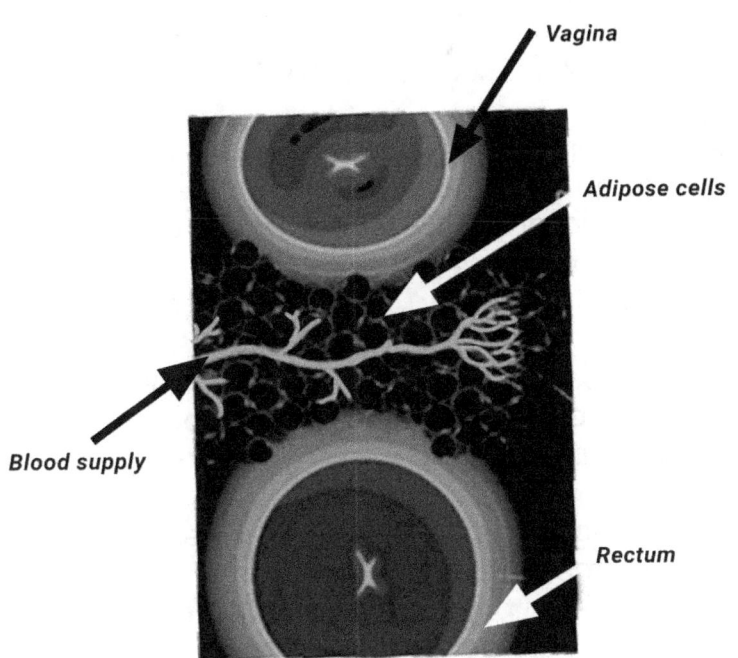

Vagina

Adipose cells

Blood supply

Rectum

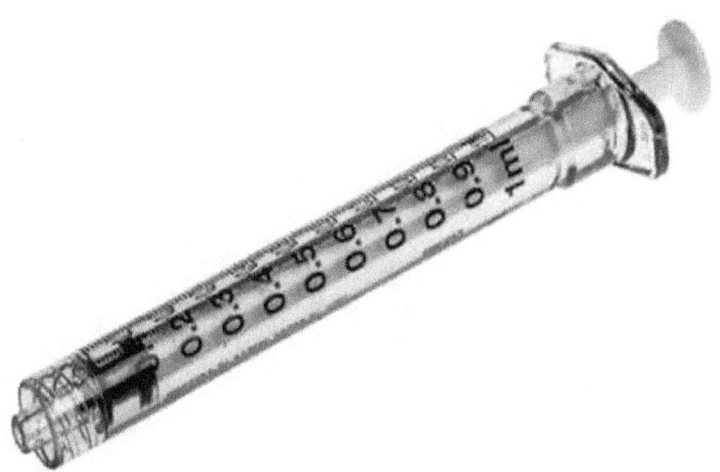

Luer lock syringe for maritus flap you can move the syringe in the middle between rectum and vagina

Episiotomy and Oasis

Medial or lateral episiotomy leads to less anal sphincter injuries than no episiotomy or midline episiotomy. The angle of episiotomy affects the occurrence of OASIS.

Perineal trauma may occur spontaneously during vaginal birth or as a result of a surgical incision (episiotomy), which is intentionally made to facilitate delivery. It is also possible to have both an episiotomy and a spontaneous tear.

Midwives and doctors that had been supervised for at least 10 mediolateral episiotomy procedures prior to independent practice knew that a mediolateral episiotomy should be performed at 60° from the midline; therefore, consideration should be given to making supervised practice mandatory, to minimize risks to pregnant people.

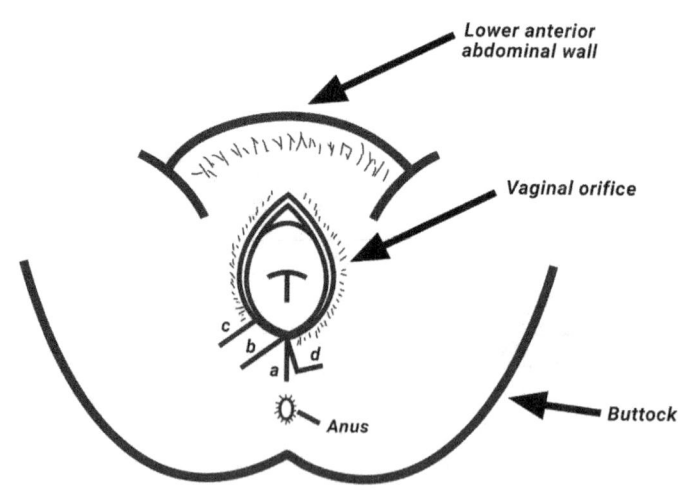

Type of Episiotomy

a: Median   b: Mediolateral   c: Transverse   d: J-shaped

Risk of complication is around 5-10 %, the risk includes abscess formation, infection, painful intercourse, or bowel incontinence.

Very rarely a connection can form between vagina and rectum (RectoVaginal fistula). It is important to report any unexpected leakage of foreign material from the vagina.

Short term perineal pain is associated with edema and bruising, in long term patients may have dyspareunia and altered sexual dysfunction.

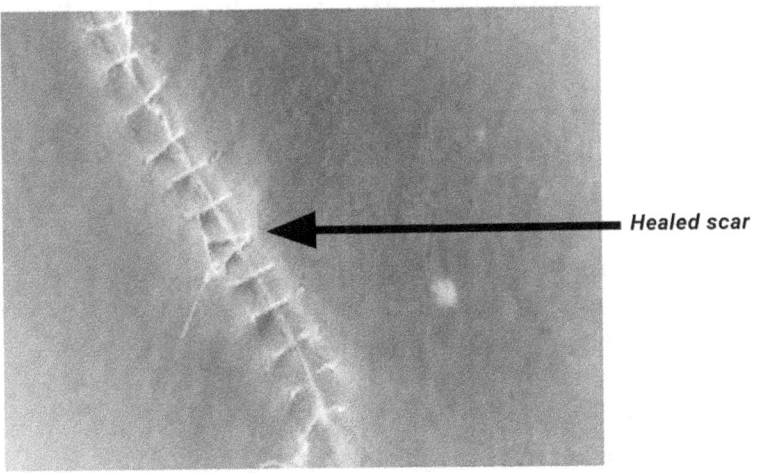

Healed scar

Repair following episiotomy incision

» Antibiotic treatment is recommended which is safe during breastfeeding, physiotherapy and pelvic floor exercises are recommended throughout the postnatal period.

» In post op appointments average 6 weeks additional information related to the healing process as well as any bowel symptoms is further evaluated.

» Eat plenty of foods containing fibers such as brown rice, cereals and fruits.

» Avoid prolonged sitting and to lie on your side

» Avoid use of bubble bath as it can delay the healing process

» Laxatives are associated with earlier and less painful first bowel motions and earlier discharge from hospital.

» Specialist endoanal ultrasound is also recommended in selective cases for evaluation incontinence to flatus or feces usually settle down in 2-3 weeks

» Endoanal ultrasonographic results have demonstrated that clinically occult anal sphincter damage during vaginal delivery is common.

» sonographic abnormalities of the anal sphincter anatomy have been identified in up to 36% of women after vaginal delivery, in prospective studies

» In 1994, Sultan et al. first described transvaginal endosonography to image the anal sphincters at rest with a rotating probe

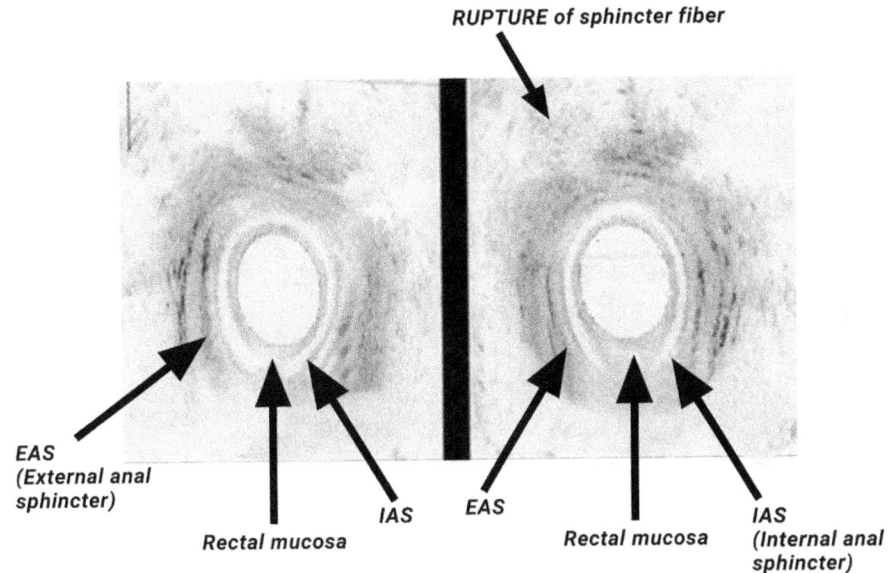

RUPTURE of sphincter fiber

EAS
(External anal
sphincter)

Rectal mucosa

IAS

EAS

Rectal mucosa

IAS
(Internal anal
sphincter)

Ultrasonic view of damaged sphincter fibers

EAS.....Showing External Anal Sphincter The external anal sphincter usually appears hyperechoic, but has a heterogeneous appearance.

IAS ..... Sowing Internal Anal Sphincter. The internal anal sphincter is a thickened continuation of the circular smooth muscle layer of the bowel and appears homogeneously hypoechoic. The development of anal endosonography added a new dimension to understanding the pathogenesis of anal incontinence and the diagnosis of obstetric anal sphincter injuries.

An endoanal ultrasound is used to demonstrate either childbirth trauma or post surgical trauma to the sphincter.

This is a muscle that maintains constriction of a natural body passage, such as the anus.

It may also show abnormal thinning of an intact internal sphincter, associated with incontinence.

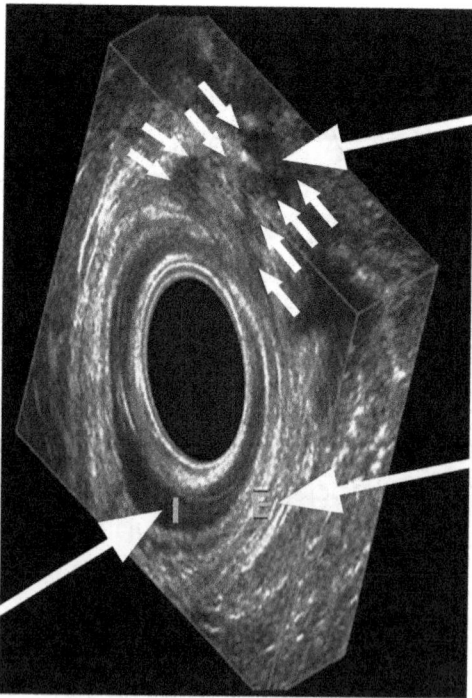

Arrows pointing towards sphinter fiber damage

E-External

I-Internal

The proximal and distal end of button hole tear must be clearly visualized. The rectal mucosa should be suture with continuous 3-0 Vicryl/PDS. The rectovaginal fascia should then be closed in layers using 2-0 Vicryl. Vaginal skin should then be closed with 2-0 Vicryl. The opinion of a colorectal surgeon is vital if there is any doubt particularly if the button hole is high (beyond) 7 cm from anal verge.

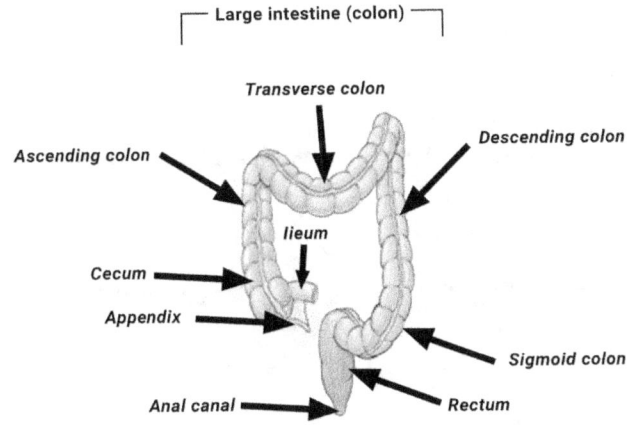

Large intestine (colon)
Transverse colon
Descending colon
Ascending colon
Ilieum
Cecum
Appendix
Sigmoid colon
Anal canal
Rectum

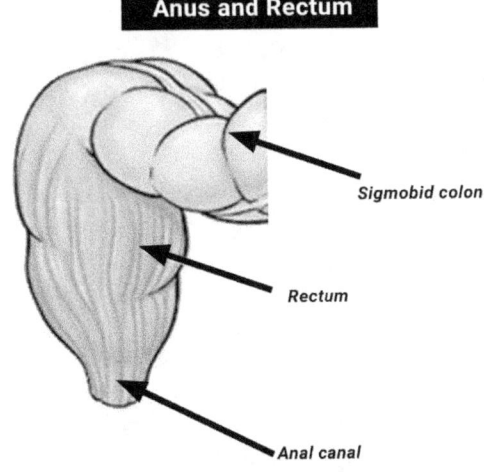

Anus and Rectum

Sigmobid colon
Rectum
Anal canal

Button Hole Injury of Rectum

Repair is performed using continuous Vicryl 3-0 Suture

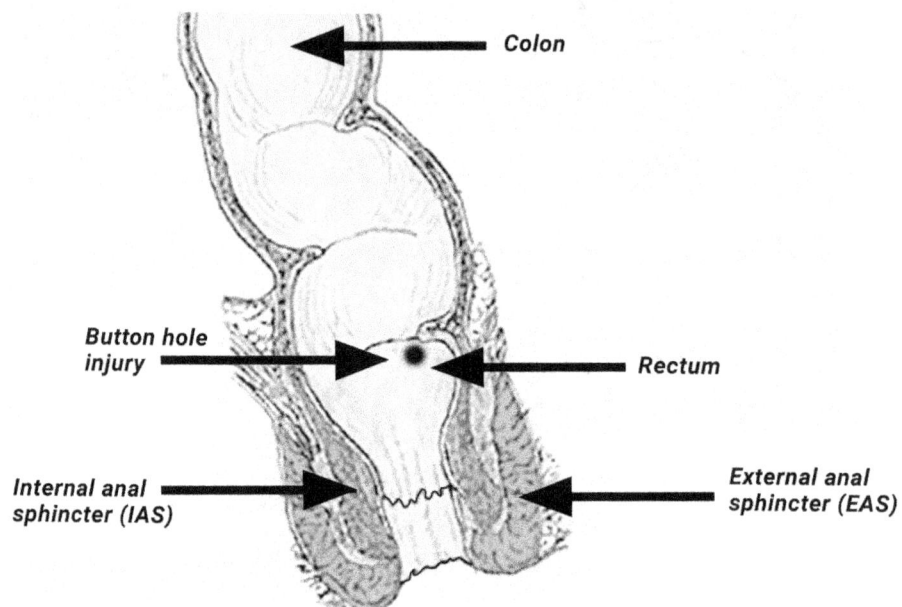

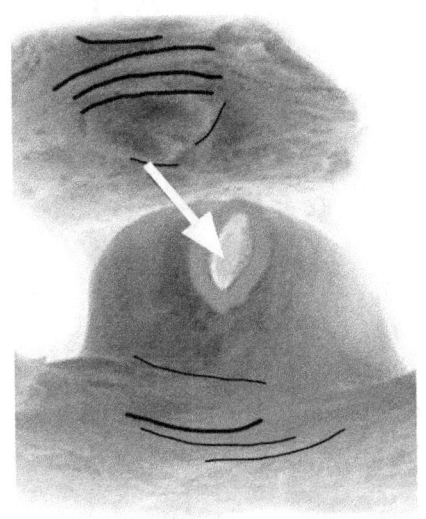

Button hole injury

The overall risk of another third or fourth degree tear with further deliveries can be 5-7%. A further advice to these women is to discuss the option in antenatal clinics to consider elective planned C/Section. (cesarean section)

Factors increasing Obstetric Anal Sphincter injury (OASI)

Certain factors increase the chance of perineal tear these include.

Shoulder Dystocia (when one of baby shoulder become stuck behind pubic bone), large baby, ethnicity (Asian and Black), epidural, prolonged pushing; persistent occipitoposterior position; nulliparity; induction of labor; epidural anesthesia; prolonged second stage >1 hour, midline episiotomy and forceps delivery.

Pelvic Floor Exercises

Pelvic floor muscle exercises involve slowly tightening and pulling up the muscle around anus and vagina. The objective of exercise is to control flatus as well as stopping the flow of urine mid -stream. Squeeze and lift, tighten and lift, minimum 3 times a day, lifting up the pelvic floor. Pelvic floor exercises are recommended to improve the continence.

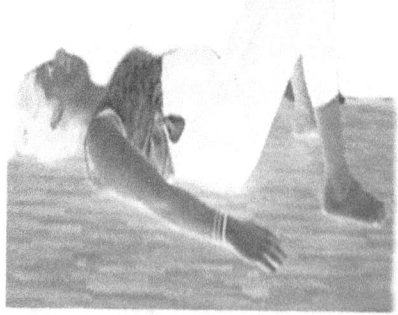
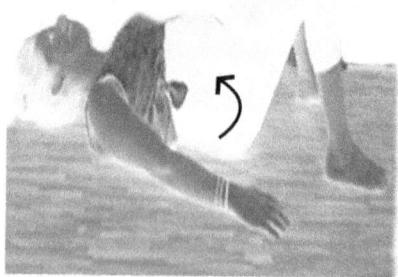

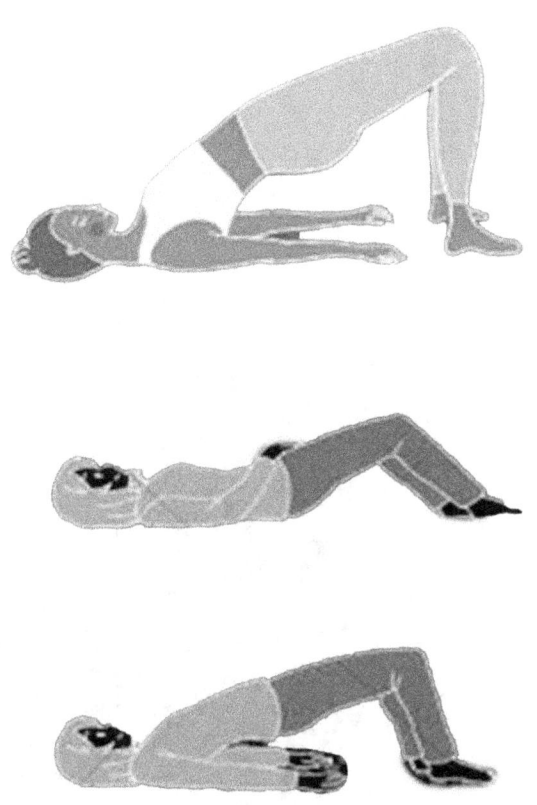

Approximately 6 weeks after the injury once vagina has healed , vaginal lubricants can be used simultaneously.

Women with third-degree tears have significantly more difficulties when doing physical exercise and in their sexual life, which is also resumed later. They more often refrain from or are hesitant about further pregnancies.

Other parameters such as mother age, breastfeeding or symptoms of pelvic floor dysfunction are additional factors influencing the resumption of coitus after delivery.

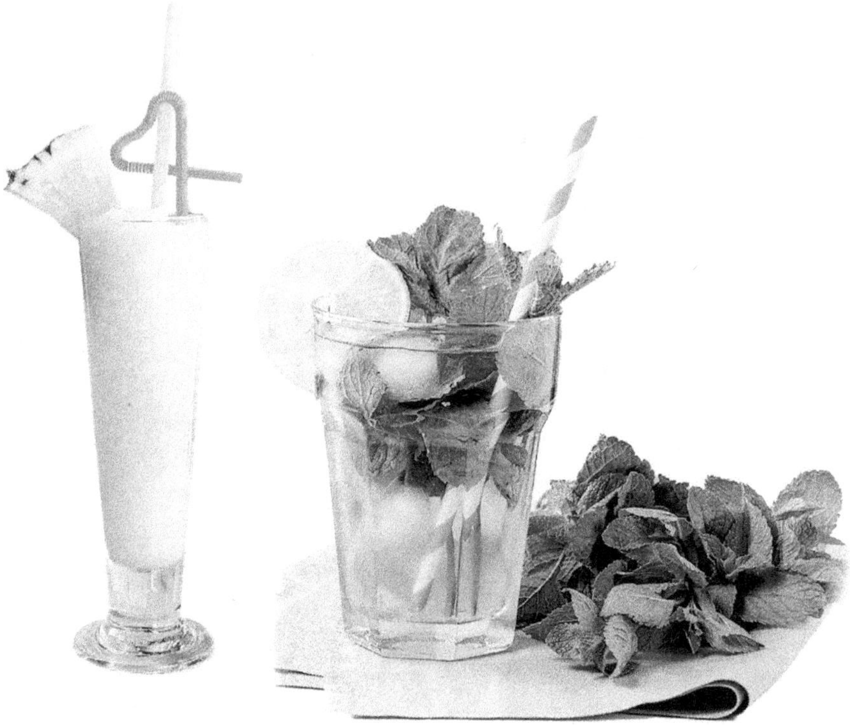

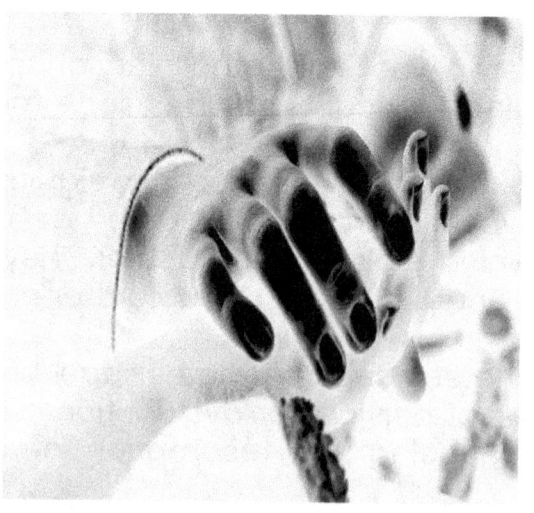

Follow up and the perineal clinic

Urogynaecology link midwives are usually involved in having questions regarding bladder or bowel symptoms. Anorectal studies are conducted 6-9 months after the delivery for some anorectal studies.

Oasis care bundle

Oasis care bundle is developed to reduce these complications during labour.

Care bundle is to enhance the patient care.

- What can be done to reduce the risk of obstetric anal sphincter injury occurring during birth.

- Manual perineal protection Women are encouraged to a slow and guided birth.

- Mediolateral Episiotomy should be performed at an angle of 60 degree from midline at crowning.

- Systemic examination of vagina and ano-rectum even if perineum is looking intact.

1. Perineal massage

2. Warm compress

3. Position: upright (using gravity) OR off you back (avoid pressure)

4. Support from midwife/obstetrician/ Colorectal/ General Surgeon/ Urogynaeclogist

5. Slow birthRest, ice, compress, elevate

6. Pain relief-Pain ladder

7. Good hygiene

8. Pelvic floor exercises

References

1. Mediolateral episiotomies: more astute decisions and fewer acute incisions https://doi.org/10.12968/bjom.2022.30.9.512

2. Anglès-Acedo, S., Ros-Cerro, C., Escura-Sancho, S. et al. Coital resumption after delivery among OASIS patients: differences between instrumental and spontaneous delivery. BMC Women's Health 19, 154

3. Okeahialam NA, Thakar R, Sultan AH. Early secondary repair of obstetric anal sphincter injuries (OASIs): experience and a review of the literature. Int Urogynecol J. 2021 Jul;32(7):1611-1622. doi: 10.1007/s00192-021-04822-x. Epub 2021 May 15. PMID: 33991222.

4. Jha S, Sultan AH. Obstetric anal sphincter injury: the changing landscape. BJOG. 2015 Jun;122(7):931. doi: 10.1111/1471-0528.13019. PMID: 26011454.

5. Okeahialam NA, Thakar R, Sultan AH. Effect of a subsequent pregnancy on anal sphincter integrity and function after obstetric anal sphincter injury (OASI). Int Urogynecol J. 2021 Jul;32(7):1719-1726. doi: 10.1007/s00192-020-04607-8. Epub 2020 Dec 2. PMID: 33263781; PMCID: PMC8295136.

6. Okeahialam NA, Sultan AH, Thakar R. The prevention of perineal trauma during vaginal birth. Am J Obstet Gynecol. 2024 Mar;230(3S):S991-S1004. doi: 10.1016/j.ajog.2022.06.021. Epub 2023 Aug 11. PMID: 37635056.

7. Fernando RJ, Sultan AH, Kettle C, Thakar R. Methods of repair for obstetric anal sphincter injury. Cochrane Database Syst Rev. 2013 Dec 8;(12):CD002866. doi: 10.1002/14651858.CD002866.pub3. PMID: 24318732.

8. Eccles A, Parsons J, Bick D, Keighley MRB, Clements A, Cornish J, Embleton S, McNiven A, Seers K, Hillman S. The GP's role in supporting women with anal incontinence after childbirth injury. Br J Gen Pract. 2024 Feb 15:BJGP.2023.0356. doi: 10.3399/BJGP.2023.0356. Epub ahead of print. PMID: 38359950.

9. Evangelopoulos N, Duraes M, Cayrac M, Galtier F, Fritel X, Gachon B, De Tayrac R. Episiotomy practice in France and prevention of high-grade perineal tears at the time of operative vaginal delivery: a prospective multicentre ancillary cohort study. Int Urogynecol J. 2024 Feb;35(2):319-326. doi: 10.1007/s00192-023-05640-z. Epub 2023 Sep 1. PMID: 37656195.

10. Orlando A, Thomas G, Murphy J, Hotouras A, Bassett P, Vaizey C. A systematic review and a meta-analysis on the incidence of obstetric anal sphincter injuries during vaginal delivery. Colorectal Dis. 2024 Feb;26(2):227-242. doi: 10.1111/codi.16831. Epub 2023 Dec 22. PMID: 38131640.

11. Mohd Raihan FS, Kusuma J, Nasution AA. Neonatal head circumference as a risk factor for obstetric anal sphincter injuries: a systematic review and meta-analysis. Am J Obstet Gynecol MFM. 2023 Aug;5(8):101047. doi: 10.1016/j.ajog mf.2023.101047. Epub 2023 Jun 3. PMID: 37277090.

12. Park M, Wanigaratne S, D'Souza R, Geoffrion R, Williams S, Muraca GM. Asian-White disparities in obstetric anal sphincter injury: a systematic review and meta-analysis. AJOG Glob Rep. 2023 Dec 10;4(1):100296. doi: 10.1016/j.xagr.2023.100296. PMID: 38283323; PMCID: PMC10820309.

13. Packet B, Page AS, Cattani L, Bosteels J, Deprest J, Richter J. Predictive factors for obstetric anal sphincter injury in primiparous women: systematic review and

meta-analysis. Ultrasound Obstet Gynecol. 2023 Oct;62(4):486-496. doi: 10.1002/uog.26292. PMID: 37329513.

14. Doxford-Hook EA, Slemeck E, Downey CL, Marsh FA. Management of levator ani avulsion: a systematic review and narrative synthesis. Arch Gynecol Obstet. 2023 Nov;308(5):1399-1408. doi: 10.1007/s00404-023-06955-4. Epub 2023 Feb 21. PMID: 36808288.

15. Woon Wong K, Okeahialam N, Thakar R, Sultan AH. Obstetric risk factors for levator ani muscle avulsion: A systematic review and meta-analysis. Eur J Obstet Gynecol Reprod Biol. 2024 May;296:99-106. doi: 10.1016/j.ejogrb.2024.02.044. Epub 2024 Feb 24. PMID: 38422805.

16. Roper JC, Thakar R, Sultan AH. UK survey of colorectal surgeons on the management of acute obstetric anal sphincter injuries. Colorectal Dis. 2024 Jan;26(1):130-136. doi: 10.1111/codi.16820. Epub 2023 Dec 26. PMID: 38148521.

17. DeLancey JOL, Masteling M, Pipitone F, LaCross J, Mastrovito S, Ashton-Miller JA. Pelvic floor injury during vaginal birth is life-altering and preventable: what can we do about it? Am J Obstet Gynecol. 2024 Mar;230(3):279-294.e2. doi: 10.1016/j.ajog.2023.11.1253. Epub 2024 Jan 2. PMID: 38168908.

18. Ramphal SR, Sultan AH. Perineal injuries during vaginal birth in low-resource countries. Best Pract Res Clin Obstet Gynaecol. 2024 Feb 15;94:102484. doi: 10.1016/j.bpobgyn.2024.102484. Epub ahead of print. PMID: 38422604.